FIBROMYALGIA DIET COOKBOOK

Mary Dixon

TABLE OF CONTENT

CHAPTER ONE

Types, Causes and Symptoms of Fibromyalgia

Fibromyalgia is a complex and often misunderstood chronic pain condition that affects millions of people worldwide. It is characterized by widespread musculoskeletal pain, tenderness, and a range of other symptoms that can significantly impact a person's quality of life.

While the exact cause of fibromyalgia remains unclear, it is believed to be a combination of genetic, environmental, and physiological factors. In this overview, we will explore the different types, potential causes, and common symptoms of fibromyalgia.

Types of Fibromyalgia:

Fibromyalgia primarily presents as one type, but there are certain variations and overlapping conditions that can occur alongside it. These include:

1. Primary Fibromyalgia: This is the most common type, where fibromyalgia exists as a standalone condition, unrelated to any other underlying health issue.

2. Secondary Fibromyalgia: Sometimes, fibromyalgia can develop secondary to another health condition, such as rheumatoid arthritis, lupus, or spinal disorders.

Causes of Fibromyalgia:

The exact cause of fibromyalgia is still not fully understood, but several factors are believed to contribute to its development:

1. Genetics: There is evidence to suggest that fibromyalgia can run in families, indicating a genetic predisposition.

2. Central Nervous System Abnormalities: Some researchers believe that abnormalities in the central nervous system's pain processing pathways can lead to heightened sensitivity to pain.

3. Physical or Emotional Trauma: Physical injuries, surgeries, or significant emotional stressors may trigger or exacerbate fibromyalgia symptoms in some individuals.

4. Infections: Certain infections, such as the Epstein-Barr virus, have been linked to the onset of fibromyalgia in some cases.

Common Symptoms of Fibromyalgia:

Fibromyalgia is characterized by a wide range of symptoms, which can vary in intensity and duration among individuals. Common symptoms include:

1. Widespread Pain: The hallmark symptom is chronic, widespread pain that affects multiple areas of the body, including muscles, tendons, and ligaments.

2. Fatigue: People with fibromyalgia often experience profound fatigue, which can be debilitating and unrelenting.

3. Sleep Disturbances: Sleep problems, including insomnia and non-restorative sleep, are common in fibromyalgia.

4. Cognitive Issues: Known as "fibro fog," this includes memory problems, difficulty concentrating, and mental confusion.

5. Morning Stiffness: Many individuals with fibromyalgia wake up feeling stiff and achy, which can improve as the day progresses.

6. Headaches: Frequent tension headaches and migraines are often associated with fibromyalgia.

7. Irritable Bowel Syndrome (IBS): Some individuals with fibromyalgia also experience digestive issues like IBS, which can include abdominal pain, diarrhea, or constipation.

8. Depression and Anxiety: Fibromyalgia can lead to mood disorders, such as depression and anxiety, often as a result of dealing with chronic pain and fatigue.

9. Sensitivity to Stimuli: Heightened sensitivity to light, noise, temperature, and touch is common, known as allodynia and hyperalgesia.

10. Muscle Stiffness and Spasms: Muscles may feel tight, and spasms or twitching can occur.

It's important to note that fibromyalgia is a highly individualized condition, and not everyone will experience all these symptoms.

Diagnosis and management typically involve a multidisciplinary approach, including a rheumatologist, pain specialist, and other healthcare providers, as well as lifestyle changes, physical therapy, and medications tailored to each patient's needs.

Fibromyalgia Diet and Benefits

Following a fibromyalgia diet can be beneficial for managing symptoms and improving overall well-being. While there is no one-size-fits-all approach, here are some general guidelines to help you get started with a fibromyalgia-friendly diet:

1. Focus on Whole Foods: Emphasize a diet rich in whole, unprocessed foods like fruits, vegetables, whole grains, lean proteins, and healthy fats. These foods provide essential nutrients and help reduce inflammation.

2. Anti-Inflammatory Foods: Include foods with anti-inflammatory properties, such as fatty fish (like salmon and mackerel), nuts, seeds, and olive oil. These can help reduce pain and inflammation.

3. Eliminate Trigger Foods: Some individuals with fibromyalgia find relief by identifying and eliminating trigger foods. Common culprits include caffeine, alcohol, artificial sweeteners, and processed foods.

4. Balanced Meals: Strive for balanced meals that include a combination of protein, carbohydrates, and healthy fats to help stabilize blood sugar levels and maintain energy.

5. Hydration: Stay well-hydrated by drinking plenty of water throughout the day. Dehydration can exacerbate symptoms like fatigue and muscle stiffness.

6. Omega-3 Fatty Acids: Incorporate omega-3-rich foods like flaxseeds, chia seeds, and walnuts, or consider fish oil supplements. Omega-3s have anti-inflammatory properties.

7. Small, Frequent Meals: Eating smaller, more frequent meals can help maintain stable blood sugar levels and prevent energy crashes.

8. Limit Processed Sugar: Minimize your intake of added sugars, as they can contribute to inflammation and energy fluctuations.

9. Monitor Food Sensitivities: Some people with fibromyalgia have food sensitivities that can worsen their symptoms. Consider working with a healthcare provider to identify and manage these sensitivities through an elimination diet or testing.

10. Avoid MSG and Aspartame: Some individuals with fibromyalgia report increased symptoms when consuming foods containing monosodium glutamate (MSG) or aspartame (an artificial sweetener). Be mindful of these ingredients.

11. Keep a Food Journal: Track your diet and symptoms in a food journal to identify patterns and potential triggers. This can help you make informed dietary choices.

12. Consult a Healthcare Provider: Always consult with a healthcare provider or registered dietitian before making significant dietary changes. They can provide personalized recommendations based on your specific needs and health status.

13. Manage Stress: Stress can exacerbate fibromyalgia symptoms. Incorporate stress-reduction techniques such as mindfulness, meditation, or yoga into your daily routine to help manage stress levels.

14. Adequate Protein Intake: Ensure you are getting enough protein from sources like lean meats, poultry, fish, tofu, or plant-based options to support muscle health.

15. Supplements: Talk to your healthcare provider about whether specific supplements like vitamin D, magnesium, or coenzyme Q10 may be beneficial for you. These can address potential deficiencies common in people with fibromyalgia.

Remember that individual responses to dietary changes can vary, so it's essential to be patient and make adjustments based on your own experiences.

A fibromyalgia diet is just one aspect of managing the condition, and it should be part of a comprehensive approach that includes medical treatment, exercise, and stress management techniques to optimize your overall health and well-being.

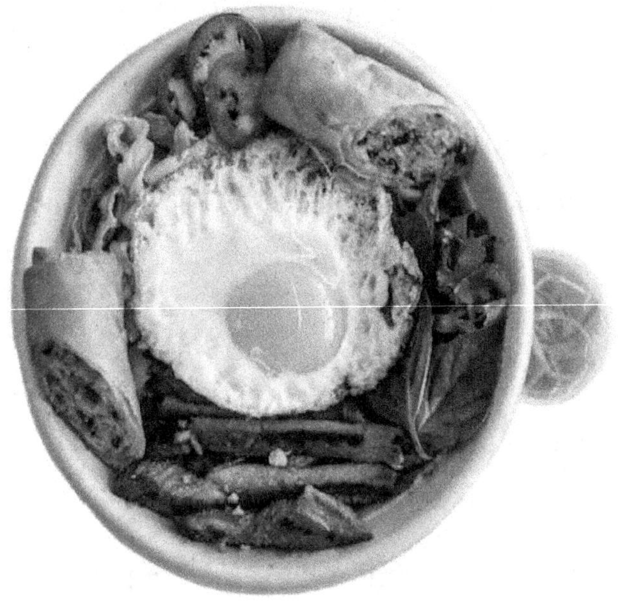

CHAPTER TWO

14-Day Fibromyalgia Diet Meal Plan

Creating a comprehensive 14-day fibromyalgia diet meal plan involves incorporating foods that are known for their potential anti-inflammatory properties and ensuring a balanced intake of essential nutrients. It's essential to remember that individual responses to food can vary, so adapt this meal plan to your specific preferences and dietary needs. Consult with a healthcare provider or a registered dietitian before making significant dietary changes.

Day 1:

- Breakfast: Oatmeal topped with fresh berries and a sprinkle of flaxseeds. A cup of green tea.
- Lunch: Grilled chicken salad with mixed greens, cherry tomatoes, cucumber, and olive oil vinaigrette.
- Dinner: Baked salmon with quinoa and steamed broccoli. Sliced strawberries for dessert.

Day 2:

- Breakfast: Greek yogurt with honey and chopped walnuts. Sliced banana on the side.

- Lunch: Lentil soup with a side of mixed greens and a whole-grain roll.
- Dinner: Stir-fried tofu with a variety of colorful vegetables in a ginger-garlic sauce, served with brown rice.

Day 3:

- Breakfast: Scrambled eggs with spinach and tomatoes. Whole-grain toast and a small glass of orange juice.
- Lunch: Turkey and avocado wrap with whole-grain tortilla and a side of carrot sticks.
- Dinner: Grilled shrimp with quinoa and roasted asparagus. A fresh fruit salad for dessert.

Day 4:

- Breakfast: Smoothie with kale, banana, almond milk, and a tablespoon of chia seeds.
- Lunch: Quinoa salad with chickpeas, roasted red peppers, and feta cheese. A drizzle of olive oil and lemon juice.
- Dinner: Baked chicken breast with sweet potato and steamed green beans.

Day 5:

- Breakfast: Cottage cheese with sliced peaches and a sprinkle of sunflower seeds.
- Lunch: Spinach and strawberry salad with grilled chicken and a balsamic vinaigrette dressing.
- Dinner: Baked cod with a quinoa and vegetable medley. A side of steamed Brussels sprouts.

Day 6:

- Breakfast: Whole-grain waffles with almond butter and sliced strawberries.
- Lunch: Turkey and vegetable stir-fry with brown rice.
- Dinner: Grilled portobello mushrooms with a spinach and pine nut stuffing. A side of roasted butternut squash.

Day 7:

- Breakfast: Smoothie bowl with acai, mixed berries, granola, and a drizzle of honey.
- Lunch: Minestrone soup with a side of mixed greens and a whole-grain roll.

- Dinner: Baked trout with quinoa and sautéed spinach. Fresh fruit salad for dessert.

Day 8:

- Breakfast: Scrambled eggs with sautéed spinach and feta cheese. Whole-grain toast and a cup of herbal tea.
- Lunch: Quinoa and black bean salad with diced tomatoes, corn, and cilantro. Drizzle with lime vinaigrette.
- Dinner: Grilled chicken breast with brown rice and steamed broccoli. A small serving of mixed berries for dessert.

Day 9:

- Breakfast: Overnight oats with almond milk, sliced almonds, and chopped apricots.
- Lunch: Mediterranean-style salad with mixed greens, cucumber, olives, cherry tomatoes, and grilled shrimp. Dress with olive oil and lemon juice.
- Dinner: Baked tilapia with a side of quinoa and roasted Brussels sprouts.

Day 10:

- Breakfast: Smoothie with spinach, banana, almond butter, and a scoop of protein powder.
- Lunch: Whole-grain wrap with hummus, roasted red peppers, cucumber, and grilled chicken strips.
- Dinner: Vegetable curry with chickpeas and brown rice. Sliced mango for dessert.

Day 11:

- Breakfast: Cottage cheese with fresh pineapple and a sprinkle of chopped pecans.
- Lunch: Spinach and feta stuffed chicken breast with a side of quinoa and sautéed green beans.
- Dinner: Baked cod with a quinoa and vegetable medley. Steamed asparagus on the side.

Day 12:

- Breakfast: Whole-grain pancakes with Greek yogurt and mixed berries.
- Lunch: Lentil and vegetable stir-fry with tofu. Serve with brown rice.

- Dinner: Grilled pork tenderloin with sweet potato
  mash and steamed broccoli. A small serving of sliced
  strawberries for dessert.

Day 13:

- Breakfast: Scrambled eggs with diced tomatoes,
  onions, and a sprinkle of cheddar cheese. Whole-
  grain toast.
- Lunch: Turkey and vegetable soup with a side of
  mixed greens and whole-grain crackers.
- Dinner: Grilled salmon with quinoa and roasted
  asparagus. A fruit salad with a drizzle of honey for
  dessert.

Day 14:

- Breakfast: Smoothie bowl with mango, kiwi,
  coconut flakes, and a handful of mixed nuts.
- Lunch: Chickpea and vegetable curry with brown
  rice.
- Dinner: Baked chicken thighs with a side of quinoa
  and sautéed spinach. Fresh fruit salad for dessert.

CHAPTER THREE

Fibromyalgia Diet Breakfast Recipes

Starting your day with a fibromyalgia-friendly breakfast can help provide sustained energy and manage symptoms. These breakfast recipes are designed to be nutritious, delicious, and suitable for individuals with fibromyalgia.

1. Berry Breakfast Parfait

Ingredients:

- 1/2 cup Greek yogurt
- 1/2 cup mixed berries (blueberries, strawberries, raspberries)
- 1 tablespoon honey or maple syrup
- 2 tablespoons granola
- A sprinkle of chopped nuts (almonds or walnuts)

Instructions:

1. In a glass or bowl, layer Greek yogurt at the bottom.

2. Add mixed berries on top of the yogurt.

3. Drizzle honey or maple syrup over the berries.

4. Sprinkle granola and chopped nuts.

5. Serve immediately.

Cooking Time: 5 minutes

2. Oatmeal with Almond Butter and Banana

Ingredients:

- 1/2 cup rolled oats
- 1 cup almond milk
- 1 ripe banana, sliced
- 1 tablespoon almond butter
- 1 teaspoon honey or maple syrup
- A pinch of cinnamon

Instructions:

1. In a saucepan, combine rolled oats and almond milk.

2. Cook over medium heat, stirring occasionally, until the oats are creamy (about 5 minutes).

3. Transfer the cooked oatmeal to a bowl.

4. Top with banana slices, almond butter, honey or maple syrup, and a pinch of cinnamon.

5. Enjoy!

Cooking Time: 10 minutes

3. Spinach and Feta Breakfast Wrap

Ingredients:

- 2 large eggs
- 1 whole-grain tortilla
- Handful of fresh spinach leaves
- 2 tablespoons crumbled feta cheese
- Salt and pepper to taste

Instructions:

1. Whisk the eggs in a bowl and season with salt and pepper.

2. Heat a non-stick skillet over medium heat and spray with cooking spray.

3. Pour the whisked eggs into the skillet and scramble until cooked.

4. Lay the tortilla flat and place the cooked eggs, fresh spinach, and feta cheese in the center.

5. Roll up the tortilla, tucking in the sides as you go.

6. Cut in half and serve.

Cooking Time: 10 minutes

4. Chia Seed Pudding with Mango

Ingredients:

- 3 tablespoons chia seeds
- 1 cup almond milk
- 1/2 cup diced mango
- 1 tablespoon honey or maple syrup
- A dash of vanilla extract

Instructions:

1. In a bowl, combine chia seeds and almond milk. Add honey or maple syrup and vanilla extract. Stir well.

2. Refrigerate for at least 2 hours or overnight, stirring occasionally until it thickens.

3. Top with diced mango before serving.

Cooking Time: 2 hours (plus chilling time)

5. Quinoa Breakfast Bowl

Ingredients:

- 1/2 cup cooked quinoa
- 1/4 cup Greek yogurt
- 1/4 cup mixed berries

- 1 tablespoon honey

- A sprinkle of chopped nuts (e.g., almonds or pecans)

Instructions:

1. In a bowl, combine cooked quinoa and Greek yogurt.

2. Top with mixed berries, drizzle honey over the top, and sprinkle with chopped nuts.

3. Serve warm or cold.

Cooking Time: 15 minutes (if quinoa is not precooked)

6. Avocado and Poached Egg Toast

Ingredients:

- 1 whole-grain toast
- 1/2 ripe avocado, mashed
- 1 poached egg
- Salt and pepper to taste
- A sprinkle of paprika (optional)

Instructions:

1. Toast the whole-grain bread.

2. Spread mashed avocado on the toast.

3. Place the poached egg on top.

4. Season with salt, pepper, and a sprinkle of paprika if desired.

Cooking Time: 15 minutes (including egg poaching)

7. Blueberry Banana Smoothie

Ingredients:

- 1 ripe banana
- 1/2 cup frozen blueberries
- 1/2 cup Greek yogurt
- 1/2 cup almond milk
- 1 tablespoon honey or maple syrup
- A handful of ice cubes

Instructions:

1. Place all ingredients in a blender.

2. Blend until smooth.

3. Pour into a glass and enjoy.

Cooking Time: 5 minutes

8. Sweet Potato Hash

Ingredients:

- 1 small sweet potato, diced
- 1/4 cup diced bell peppers
- 1/4 cup diced onions
- 1/4 cup cooked and crumbled turkey sausage (optional)
- 1 tablespoon olive oil
- Salt and pepper to taste

Instructions:

1. Heat olive oil in a skillet over medium heat.

2. Add sweet potato, bell peppers, and onions. Sauté until sweet potatoes are tender and slightly crispy.

3. Add cooked turkey sausage (if using) and season with salt and pepper.

4. Serve hot.

Cooking Time: 20 minutes

9. Apple Cinnamon Quinoa Bowl

Ingredients:

- 1/2 cup cooked quinoa
- 1/2 apple, diced
- 1/2 teaspoon cinnamon
- 1 tablespoon almond butter
- 1 teaspoon honey or maple syrup

Instructions:

1. In a bowl, combine cooked quinoa, diced apple, and cinnamon.

2. Drizzle almond butter and honey or maple syrup over the top.

3. Mix well and enjoy.

Cooking Time: 15 minutes (if quinoa is not precooked)

10. Veggie Omelette

Ingredients:

- 2 large eggs
- 1/4 cup diced bell peppers
- 1/4 cup diced onions

- 1/4 cup diced tomatoes

- 1/4 cup chopped spinach

- 1 tablespoon olive oil

- Salt and pepper to taste

Instructions:

1. In a bowl, whisk the eggs and season with salt and pepper.

2. Heat olive oil in a non-stick skillet over medium heat.

3. Add bell peppers, onions, and tomatoes. Sauté until softened.

4. Pour the whisked eggs over the sautéed vegetables.

5. Cook until the omelette sets, then fold it in half.

6. Slide onto a plate and serve.

Cooking Time: 10 minutes

Fibromyalgia Diet Lunch Recipes

1. Quinoa and Chickpea Salad

This protein-packed salad is loaded with fiber, vitamins, and minerals, making it an excellent choice for a fibromyalgia-friendly lunch.

Ingredients:

- 1 cup cooked quinoa
- 1 can (15 oz) chickpeas, drained and rinsed
- 1 cucumber, diced
- 1 red bell pepper, diced
- 1/4 cup fresh parsley, chopped
- Juice of 1 lemon
- 2 tablespoons olive oil
- Salt and pepper to taste

Instructions:

1. In a large bowl, combine quinoa, chickpeas, cucumber, red bell pepper, and fresh parsley.

2. Drizzle with lemon juice and olive oil, then season with salt and pepper.

3. Toss to combine and serve.

Cooking Time: 20 minutes (if quinoa is not precooked)

2. Spinach and Quinoa Stuffed Bell Peppers

These stuffed bell peppers are filled with nutrient-rich ingredients, providing a satisfying and fibromyalgia-friendly lunch option.

Ingredients:

- 4 bell peppers (any color)
- 1 cup cooked quinoa
- 1 cup chopped spinach
- 1/2 cup diced tomatoes
- 1/2 cup black beans, drained and rinsed
- 1/2 cup corn kernels
- 1/2 teaspoon cumin
- 1/2 teaspoon chili powder
- Salt and pepper to taste
- Grated cheese (optional, for topping)

Instructions:

1. Preheat the oven to 375°F (190°C).

2. Cut the tops off the bell peppers and remove the seeds and membranes.

3. In a bowl, combine quinoa, chopped spinach, diced tomatoes, black beans, corn, cumin, chili powder, salt, and pepper.

4. Stuff the mixture into the bell peppers.

5. Place the stuffed peppers in a baking dish and cover with foil.

6. Bake for 30-35 minutes until peppers are tender.

7. If desired, sprinkle grated cheese on top and bake for an additional 5 minutes until cheese is melted.

Cooking Time: 40-45 minutes (if quinoa is not precooked)

3. Lentil and Vegetable Soup

A hearty and nutritious soup, packed with fiber and plant-based protein, perfect for a comforting and fibromyalgia-friendly lunch.

Ingredients:

- 1 cup dried green or brown lentils, rinsed and drained
- 1 onion, diced
- 2 carrots, diced
- 2 celery stalks, diced
- 1 bell pepper, diced
- 3 cloves garlic, minced
- 6 cups vegetable broth
- 1 can (14 oz) diced tomatoes
- 1 teaspoon dried thyme

- Salt and pepper to taste

Instructions:

1. In a large pot, heat some olive oil over medium heat.

2. Add onions, carrots, celery, bell pepper, and garlic. Sauté until vegetables are softened.

3. Add lentils, vegetable broth, diced tomatoes (with their juice), thyme, salt, and pepper.

4. Bring to a boil, then reduce heat, cover, and simmer for about 30-35 minutes until lentils are tender.

5. Adjust seasoning as needed and serve.

Cooking Time: 45-50 minutes

4. Turkey and Avocado Wrap

A simple and satisfying wrap filled with lean protein and healthy fats, perfect for a quick and fibromyalgia-friendly lunch.

Ingredients:

- 1 whole-grain tortilla
- 4-6 slices of roasted turkey breast

- 1/2 avocado, sliced

- 1/4 cup mixed greens

- 1 tablespoon hummus or Greek yogurt dressing

Instructions:

1. Lay the whole-grain tortilla flat.

2. Place the turkey slices on the tortilla.

3. Add sliced avocado, mixed greens, and a drizzle of hummus or Greek yogurt dressing.

4. Roll up the tortilla, tucking in the sides as you go.

5. Cut in half and serve.

Cooking Time: 10 minutes (if turkey is not precooked)

5. Mediterranean Chickpea Salad

This Mediterranean-inspired salad is rich in flavor and nutrients, featuring ingredients known for their potential anti-inflammatory benefits.

Ingredients:

- 1 can (15 oz) chickpeas, drained and rinsed

- 1 cucumber, diced

- 1 cup cherry tomatoes, halved
- 1/4 cup Kalamata olives, pitted and chopped
- 1/4 cup red onion, finely chopped
- 1/4 cup crumbled feta cheese
- Juice of 1 lemon
- 2 tablespoons extra-virgin olive oil
- 1 teaspoon dried oregano
- Salt and pepper to taste

Instructions:

1. In a large bowl, combine chickpeas, cucumber, cherry tomatoes, Kalamata olives, red onion, and feta cheese.

2. Drizzle with lemon juice and olive oil, then sprinkle with dried oregano, salt, and pepper.

3. Toss to combine and serve.

Cooking Time: 15 minutes

6. Tuna and White Bean Salad

A protein-packed salad featuring tuna and white beans, known for their omega-3 fatty acids and fiber content, making it suitable for a fibromyalgia-friendly lunch.

Ingredients:

- 1 can (5 oz) tuna, drained
- 1 can (15 oz) cannellini or white beans, drained and rinsed
- 1/4 cup diced red onion
- 1/4 cup diced celery
- 1/4 cup diced red bell pepper
- 2 tablespoons chopped fresh parsley
- Juice of 1 lemon
- 2 tablespoons olive oil
- Salt and pepper to taste

Instructions:

1. In a bowl, combine tuna, white beans, red onion, celery, red bell pepper, and fresh parsley.

2. Drizzle with lemon juice and olive oil, then season with salt and pepper.

3. Mix well and serve.

Cooking Time: 15 minutes

7. Sweet Potato and Black Bean Bowl

A satisfying and fiber-rich lunch bowl featuring sweet potatoes and black beans, known for their potential anti-inflammatory properties.

Ingredients:

- 1 medium sweet potato, diced
- 1 cup cooked black beans
- 1/2 cup corn kernels
- 1/2 avocado, sliced
- 2 tablespoons salsa
- 2 tablespoons Greek yogurt or dairy-free alternative (for topping)
- Fresh cilantro for garnish
- Salt and pepper to taste

Instructions:

1. Preheat the oven to 425°F (220°C).

2. Toss sweet potato cubes with olive oil, salt, and pepper, then spread them on a baking sheet.

3. Roast for 25-30 minutes until sweet potatoes are tender and slightly crispy.

4. In a bowl, combine cooked black beans, corn kernels, and avocado slices.

5. Top with roasted sweet potatoes, salsa, a dollop of Greek yogurt (or dairy-free alternative), and garnish with fresh cilantro.

Cooking Time: 40-45 minutes (including roasting sweet potatoes)

8. Salmon Salad with Lemon-Dill Dressing

A delicious and omega-3-rich salad featuring salmon and leafy greens, which may help reduce inflammation and manage fibromyalgia symptoms.

Ingredients:

- 2 salmon fillets
- 4 cups mixed greens
- 1/4 red onion, thinly sliced
- 1/4 cup cherry tomatoes, halved
- Juice of 1 lemon
- 2 tablespoons olive oil
- 1 tablespoon fresh dill, chopped
- Salt and pepper to taste

Instructions:

1. Season salmon fillets with salt and pepper.

2. Heat olive oil in a skillet over medium-high heat.

3. Add salmon fillets and cook for 4-5 minutes per side until cooked through.

4. In a bowl, combine mixed greens, red onion, and cherry tomatoes.

5. Whisk together lemon juice, olive oil, fresh dill, salt, and pepper to make the dressing.

6. Drizzle the dressing over the salad.

7. Top the salad with cooked salmon fillets.

Cooking Time: 15 minutes

9. Vegetable and Quinoa Stir-Fry

A nutritious stir-fry packed with colorful vegetables and protein-rich quinoa, providing a satisfying and fibromyalgia-friendly lunch option.

Ingredients:

-    1 cup cooked quinoa

- 1 cup broccoli florets
- 1 cup bell peppers (assorted colors), sliced
- 1 cup snap peas
- 1 cup carrots, sliced
- 1 cup tofu, cubed
- 2 tablespoons low-sodium soy sauce or tamari
- 1 tablespoon sesame oil
- 1 teaspoon ginger, minced
- 2 cloves garlic, minced
- Salt and pepper to taste

Instructions:

1. In a large skillet or wok, heat sesame oil over medium-high heat.

2. Add ginger and garlic, and stir-fry for about 30 seconds.

3. Add tofu and cook until lightly browned.

4. Add broccoli, bell peppers, snap peas, and carrots. Stir-fry for 4-5 minutes until vegetables are tender-crisp.

5. Add cooked quinoa, soy sauce or tamari, salt, and pepper. Stir-fry for an additional 2-3 minutes.

6. Adjust seasoning as needed and serve.

Cooking Time: 25 minutes (if quinoa is not precooked)

10. Caprese Salad with Balsamic Glaze

A classic Caprese salad with a twist—drizzled with balsamic glaze for added flavor and antioxidants.

Ingredients:

- 2 large tomatoes, sliced
- 1 cup fresh mozzarella cheese, sliced
- 1/4 cup fresh basil leaves
- 2 tablespoons extra-virgin olive oil
- Balsamic glaze for drizzling
- Salt and pepper to taste

Instructions:

1. Arrange tomato and mozzarella slices on a serving platter, alternating them.

2. Tuck fresh basil leaves between the tomato and mozzarella slices.

3. Drizzle with extra-virgin olive oil.

4. Season with salt and pepper.

5. Finish with a generous drizzle of balsamic glaze.

6. Serve chilled.

Cooking Time: 10 minutes

These lunch recipes offer a variety of options that can help you maintain a fibromyalgia-friendly diet while enjoying delicious and nutritious meals.

Adjust ingredients and portion sizes according to your preferences and dietary needs.

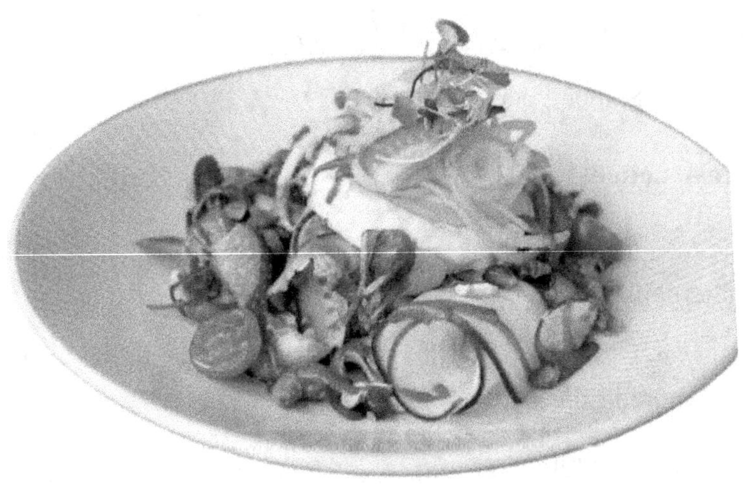

CHAPTER FOUR

Fibromyalgia Diet Dinner Recipes

1. Baked Salmon with Lemon-Dill Sauce

Salmon is rich in omega-3 fatty acids, known for their potential anti-inflammatory properties, making it an excellent choice for a fibromyalgia-friendly dinner.

Ingredients:

- 4 salmon fillets
- Juice of 1 lemon
- 2 tablespoons olive oil
- 1 tablespoon fresh dill, chopped
- Salt and pepper to taste

Instructions:

1. Preheat the oven to 375°F (190°C).

2. Place salmon fillets on a baking sheet.

3. In a bowl, whisk together lemon juice, olive oil, fresh dill, salt, and pepper.

4. Drizzle the lemon-dill sauce over the salmon fillets.

5. Bake for 15-20 minutes until the salmon flakes easily with a fork.

6. Serve hot.

Cooking Time: 20-25 minutes

2. Quinoa-Stuffed Bell Peppers

These stuffed bell peppers are filled with quinoa and vegetables, providing a satisfying and fibromyalgia-friendly dinner option.

Ingredients:

- 4 bell peppers (any color)
- 1 cup cooked quinoa
- 1/2 cup diced tomatoes
- 1/2 cup black beans, drained and rinsed
- 1/2 cup corn kernels
- 1/2 teaspoon cumin
- 1/2 teaspoon chili powder
- Salt and pepper to taste
- Grated cheese (optional, for topping)

Instructions:

1. Preheat the oven to 375°F (190°C).

2. Cut the tops off the bell peppers and remove the seeds and membranes.

3. In a bowl, combine cooked quinoa, diced tomatoes, black beans, corn, cumin, chili powder, salt, and pepper.

4. Stuff the mixture into the bell peppers.

5. Place the stuffed peppers in a baking dish and cover with foil.

6. Bake for 30-35 minutes until peppers are tender.

7. If desired, sprinkle grated cheese on top and bake for an additional 5 minutes until cheese is melted.

Cooking Time: 40-45 minutes (if quinoa is not precooked)

3. Chicken and Vegetable Stir-Fry

A flavorful stir-fry featuring lean chicken and colorful vegetables, perfect for a quick and fibromyalgia-friendly dinner.

Ingredients:

- 2 boneless, skinless chicken breasts, cut into strips
- 2 cups mixed vegetables (bell peppers, broccoli, snap peas, carrots)
- 2 cloves garlic, minced
- 1 tablespoon ginger, minced
- 2 tablespoons low-sodium soy sauce or tamari
- 1 tablespoon honey or maple syrup
- 1 tablespoon olive oil
- Salt and pepper to taste

Instructions:

1. In a small bowl, whisk together soy sauce, honey or maple syrup, garlic, and ginger.

2. Heat olive oil in a large skillet or wok over medium-high heat.

3. Add chicken strips and cook until browned and cooked through.

4. Remove chicken from the skillet.

5. In the same skillet, add mixed vegetables and stir-fry for 3-4 minutes until tender-crisp.

6. Return cooked chicken to the skillet.

7. Pour the soy sauce mixture over the chicken and vegetables.

8. Stir-fry for an additional 2-3 minutes.

9. Season with salt and pepper.

10. Serve hot.

Cooking Time: 20 minutes

4. Lentil and Vegetable Curry

A hearty and flavorful lentil and vegetable curry, rich in fiber and plant-based protein, making it an excellent choice for a fibromyalgia-friendly dinner.

Ingredients:

- 1 cup dried red or brown lentils, rinsed and drained
- 1 onion, diced
- 2 cloves garlic, minced
- 1 tablespoon ginger, minced
- 2 carrots, diced
- 2 potatoes, diced
- 1 can (14 oz) diced tomatoes

- 1 can (14 oz) coconut milk

- 2 tablespoons curry powder

- Salt and pepper to taste

Instructions:

1. In a large pot, heat some olive oil over medium heat.

2. Add onions, garlic, and ginger. Sauté until onions are translucent.

3. Add lentils, carrots, potatoes, diced tomatoes (with their juice), coconut milk, curry powder, salt, and pepper.

4. Bring to a boil, then reduce heat, cover, and simmer for about 20-25 minutes until lentils and vegetables are tender.

5. Adjust seasoning as needed and serve.

Cooking Time: 30-35 minutes

5. Sweet Potato and Black Bean Quesadillas

These quesadillas are filled with nutritious ingredients like sweet potatoes and black beans, offering a satisfying and fibromyalgia-friendly dinner option.

Ingredients:

- 2 large whole-grain tortillas
- 1 large sweet potato, diced and roasted
- 1 can (15 oz) black beans, drained and rinsed
- 1 cup shredded cheddar cheese (or dairy-free alternative)
- 1 teaspoon cumin
- 1/2 teaspoon chili powder
- Salt and pepper to taste
- Olive oil for cooking

Instructions:

1. Preheat the oven to 375°F (190°C).

2. Toss sweet potato cubes with olive oil, salt, pepper, cumin, and chili powder, then spread them on a baking sheet.

3. Roast for 25-30 minutes until sweet potatoes are tender and slightly crispy.

4. Heat a non-stick skillet over medium heat.

5. Place one tortilla in the skillet.

6. Layer one-half of the tortilla with sweet potatoes, black beans, and shredded cheese.

7. Fold the other half of the tortilla over the filling.

8. Cook until the bottom is golden brown, then flip and cook the other side.

9. Repeat with the second tortilla.

10. Cut into wedges and serve.

Cooking Time: 40-45 minutes (including roasting sweet potatoes)

6. Lemon Herb Baked Chicken

A simple and flavorful baked chicken dish with lemon and herbs, perfect for a light and fibromyalgia-friendly dinner.

Ingredients:

- 4 boneless, skinless chicken breasts
- Juice of 2 lemons
- 2 tablespoons olive oil
- 2 cloves garlic, minced
- 2 teaspoons dried oregano
- Salt and pepper to taste

- Lemon slices for garnish

Instructions:

1. Preheat the oven to 375°F (190°C).

2. In a bowl, whisk together lemon juice, olive oil, garlic, dried oregano, salt, and pepper.

3. Place chicken breasts in a baking dish.

4. Pour the lemon-herb mixture over the chicken.

5. Add lemon slices on top.

6. Bake for 25-30 minutes until the chicken is cooked through and no longer pink in the center.

7. Serve hot.

Cooking Time: 30-35 minutes

7. Vegetable and Tofu Stir-Fry

A colorful and nutritious stir-fry featuring tofu and a variety of vegetables, offering a satisfying and fibromyalgia-friendly dinner option.

Ingredients:

- 1 package (14 oz) extra-firm tofu, cubed and pressed

- 2 cups mixed vegetables (bell peppers, broccoli, snap peas, carrots)
- 2 cloves garlic, minced
- 1 tablespoon ginger, minced
- 2 tablespoons low-sodium soy sauce or tamari
- 1 tablespoon honey or maple syrup
- 1 tablespoon olive oil
- Salt and pepper to taste

Instructions:

1. In a small bowl, whisk together soy sauce, honey or maple syrup, garlic, and ginger.

2. Heat olive oil in a large skillet or wok over medium-high heat.

3. Add tofu cubes and cook until browned on all sides.

4. Remove tofu from the skillet.

5. In the same skillet, add mixed vegetables and stir-fry for 3-4 minutes until tender-crisp.

6. Return cooked tofu to the skillet.

7. Pour the soy sauce mixture over the tofu and vegetables.

8. Stir-fry for an additional 2-3 minutes.

9. Season with salt and pepper.

10. Serve hot.

Cooking Time: 20 minutes

8. Lentil and Vegetable Soup

A comforting and hearty lentil soup filled with vegetables, rich in fiber and plant-based protein, perfect for a nourishing and fibromyalgia-friendly dinner.

Ingredients:

- 1 cup dried green or brown lentils, rinsed and drained
- 1 onion, diced
- 2 carrots, diced
- 2 celery stalks, diced
- 1 bell pepper, diced
- 3 cloves garlic, minced
- 6 cups vegetable broth
- 1 can (14 oz) diced tomatoes
- 1 teaspoon dried thyme
- Salt and pepper to taste

Instructions:

1. In a large pot, heat some olive oil over medium heat.

2. Add onions, carrots, celery, bell pepper, and garlic. Sauté until vegetables are softened.

3. Add lentils, vegetable broth, diced tomatoes (with their juice), thyme, salt, and pepper.

4. Bring to a boil, then reduce heat, cover, and simmer for about 30-35 minutes until lentils are tender.

5. Adjust seasoning as needed and serve.

Cooking Time: 45-50 minutes

9. Mediterranean Chickpea Salad

A vibrant Mediterranean-inspired salad packed with fiber and flavor, making it an ideal choice for a fibromyalgia-friendly dinner.

Ingredients:

- 1 can (15 oz) chickpeas, drained and rinsed
- 1 cucumber, diced
- 1 cup cherry tomatoes, halved
- 1/4 cup Kalamata olives, pitted and chopped

- 1/4 cup red onion, finely chopped

- 1/4 cup crumbled feta cheese

- Juice of 1 lemon

- 2 tablespoons extra-virgin olive oil

- 1 teaspoon dried oregano

- Salt and pepper to taste

Instructions:

1. In a large bowl, combine chickpeas, cucumber, cherry tomatoes, Kalamata olives, red onion, and feta cheese.

2. Drizzle with lemon juice and olive oil, then sprinkle with dried oregano, salt, and pepper.

3. Toss to combine and serve.

Cooking Time: 15 minutes

10. Turkey and Vegetable Stir-Fry

A quick and wholesome turkey stir-fry with a variety of colorful vegetables, offering a flavorful and fibromyalgia-friendly dinner option.

Ingredients:

- 1 pound ground turkey

- 2 cups mixed vegetables (bell peppers, broccoli, snap peas, carrots)
- 2 cloves garlic, minced
- 1 tablespoon ginger, minced
- 2 tablespoons low-sodium soy sauce or tamari
- 1 tablespoon honey or maple syrup
- 1 tablespoon olive oil
- Salt and pepper to taste

Instructions:

1. In a small bowl, whisk together soy sauce, honey or maple syrup, garlic, and ginger.

2. Heat olive oil in a large skillet or wok over medium-high heat.

3. Add ground turkey and cook until browned and cooked through.

4. Remove turkey from the skillet.

5. In the same skillet, add mixed vegetables and stir-fry for 3-4 minutes until tender-crisp.

6. Return cooked turkey to the skillet.

7. Pour the soy sauce mixture over the turkey and vegetables.

8. Stir-fry for an additional 2-3 minutes.

9. Season with salt and pepper.

10. Serve hot.

Cooking Time: 20 minutes

Fibromyalgia Diet Snack Recipes

1. Greek Yogurt and Berry Parfait

A creamy and satisfying snack loaded with protein and antioxidants, perfect for managing fibromyalgia symptoms.

Ingredients:

- 1/2 cup Greek yogurt
- 1/2 cup mixed berries (blueberries, strawberries, raspberries)
- 1 tablespoon honey or maple syrup
- 2 tablespoons granola
- A sprinkle of chopped nuts (almonds or walnuts)

Instructions:

1. In a glass or bowl, layer Greek yogurt at the bottom.

2. Add mixed berries on top of the yogurt.

3. Drizzle honey or maple syrup over the berries.

4. Sprinkle granola and chopped nuts.

5. Serve immediately.

Cooking Time: 5 minutes

2. Hummus and Veggie Sticks

A simple and nutritious snack featuring fiber-rich vegetables and protein-packed hummus.

Ingredients:

- Assorted veggie sticks (carrots, cucumber, bell peppers, celery)
- 1/4 cup hummus

Instructions:

1. Wash and cut the veggies into sticks.

2. Serve with a side of hummus for dipping.

Cooking Time: 10 minutes (prep time)

3. Cottage Cheese with Pineapple

A protein-rich and creamy snack that combines the goodness of cottage cheese and the sweetness of pineapple.

Ingredients:

- 1/2 cup low-fat cottage cheese

- 1/2 cup diced pineapple (fresh or canned in juice)

Instructions:

1. Combine cottage cheese and diced pineapple in a bowl.

2. Mix well and enjoy.

Cooking Time: 5 minutes

4. Almond Butter and Banana Toast

A tasty and satisfying snack with the creaminess of almond butter and the sweetness of bananas.

Ingredients:

- 1 slice whole-grain bread
- 2 tablespoons almond butter
- 1/2 banana, sliced
- A drizzle of honey (optional)

Instructions:

1. Toast the whole-grain bread.

2. Spread almond butter on the toast.

3. Top with banana slices and a drizzle of honey if desired.

Cooking Time: 5 minutes

5. Chia Seed Pudding with Mango

A fiber-rich and refreshing snack featuring chia seeds and tropical mango.

Ingredients:

- 3 tablespoons chia seeds
- 1 cup almond milk
- 1/2 cup diced mango
- 1 tablespoon honey or maple syrup
- A dash of vanilla extract

Instructions:

1. In a bowl, combine chia seeds and almond milk. Add honey or maple syrup and vanilla extract. Stir well.

2. Refrigerate for at least 2 hours or overnight, stirring occasionally until it thickens.

3. Top with diced mango before serving.

Cooking Time: 2 hours (plus chilling time)

6. Mixed Nuts and Dried Fruits

A convenient and nutrient-packed snack with a variety of nuts and dried fruits.

Ingredients:

- 1/4 cup mixed nuts (almonds, walnuts, cashews)
- 1/4 cup mixed dried fruits (raisins, apricots, cranberries)

Instructions:

1. Combine mixed nuts and dried fruits in a small bowl.

2. Toss together and enjoy.

Cooking Time: 5 minutes (prep time)

7. Apple Slices with Almond Butter

A simple and satisfying snack pairing crisp apple slices with creamy almond butter.

Ingredients:

- 1 apple, sliced
- 2 tablespoons almond butter

Instructions:

1. Slice the apple into wedges.

2. Dip apple slices in almond butter and enjoy.

Cooking Time: 5 minutes (prep time)

8. Rice Cakes with Avocado and Cherry Tomatoes

A crunchy and nutritious snack combining rice cakes, creamy avocado, and cherry tomatoes.

Ingredients:

- 2 rice cakes
- 1/2 avocado, mashed
- 6-8 cherry tomatoes, halved
- A sprinkle of salt and pepper

Instructions:

1. Spread mashed avocado on each rice cake.

2. Top with cherry tomato halves.

3. Sprinkle with salt and pepper to taste.

Cooking Time: 5 minutes (prep time)

9. Roasted Chickpeas

A crunchy and protein-packed snack that's perfect for munching.

Ingredients:

- 1 can (15 oz) chickpeas, drained and rinsed
- 1 tablespoon olive oil
- 1 teaspoon paprika
- 1/2 teaspoon garlic powder
- Salt and pepper to taste

Instructions:

1. Preheat the oven to 375°F (190°C).

2. Pat chickpeas dry with a paper towel.

3. In a bowl, toss chickpeas with olive oil, paprika, garlic powder, salt, and pepper.

4. Spread chickpeas on a baking sheet.

5. Roast for 30-35 minutes until crispy, shaking the pan occasionally.

6. Let cool before enjoying.

Cooking Time: 40-45 minutes

10. Cottage Cheese and Sliced Peaches

A protein-rich and fruity snack combining cottage cheese with the sweetness of sliced peaches.

Ingredients:

- 1/2 cup low-fat cottage cheese
- 1/2 peach, sliced

Instructions:

1. Place cottage cheese in a bowl.

2. Top with sliced peaches and enjoy.

Cooking Time: 5 minutes (prep time)

These snack recipes offer a variety of choices to help you maintain a fibromyalgia-friendly diet while satisfying your cravings.

Adjust portion sizes according to your preferences and dietary needs.

CONCLUSION

Adopting a fibromyalgia diet can be a crucial step in managing this chronic condition and improving overall well-being.

Fibromyalgia is a complex disorder that involves widespread pain, fatigue, and a range of other symptoms, often accompanied by sleep disturbances and mood disorders.

While there is no cure for fibromyalgia, dietary changes can play a significant role in alleviating symptoms and enhancing the quality of life for those affected.

A fibromyalgia diet primarily focuses on incorporating nutrient-rich foods that have been associated with reduced inflammation, improved sleep, and better energy levels. This includes a variety of fruits and vegetables, lean proteins, whole grains, and healthy fats.

Antioxidant-rich foods, such as berries, leafy greens, and fatty fish, can help combat oxidative stress and inflammation, which are common features of fibromyalgia.

Additionally, maintaining stable blood sugar levels through balanced meals and snacks can help prevent energy crashes and mood swings that are often experienced by individuals with fibromyalgia.

Choosing complex carbohydrates like whole grains and legumes over refined sugars can contribute to more stable energy levels.

Moreover, it's important to stay hydrated and limit caffeine and alcohol intake, as these substances can disrupt sleep patterns and exacerbate fibromyalgia symptoms.

While a fibromyalgia diet can provide substantial relief, it is essential to personalize your approach to suit your specific needs and preferences. Consulting with a healthcare professional or registered dietitian who is knowledgeable about fibromyalgia can be highly beneficial in creating a tailored dietary plan.

In addition to dietary changes, individuals with fibromyalgia should also consider other lifestyle modifications, including stress management, regular exercise within one's capabilities, and proper sleep hygiene, as these factors can work in tandem with diet to improve overall health and well-being.

Ultimately, while fibromyalgia can be challenging to manage, a thoughtful and well-balanced diet can be a powerful tool in your arsenal against the condition.

By making mindful choices about the foods you consume and being attentive to your body's responses, you can take proactive steps to enhance your quality of life and reduce the impact of fibromyalgia symptoms.

Remember that individual responses to dietary changes may vary, so it's important to work closely with healthcare professionals to determine the most effective strategies for your unique situation.

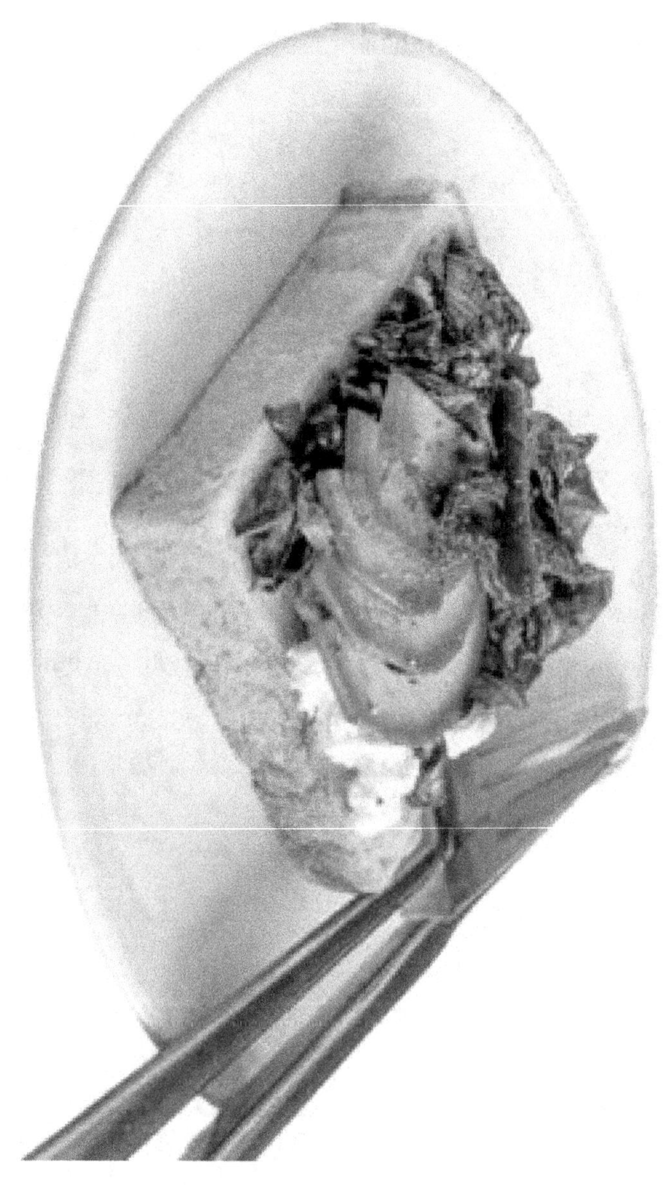

www.ingramcontent.com/pod-product-compliance
Lightning Source LLC
Chambersburg PA
CBHW050852260726
48660CB00006B/2580